The Pegan

Diet

The Pegan diet blends the ancient Paleo diet with the more modern Vegan diet.

Eating a mostly plant based diet but with meat Poultry and fish as condiments

will increase weight loss and improve heart health.

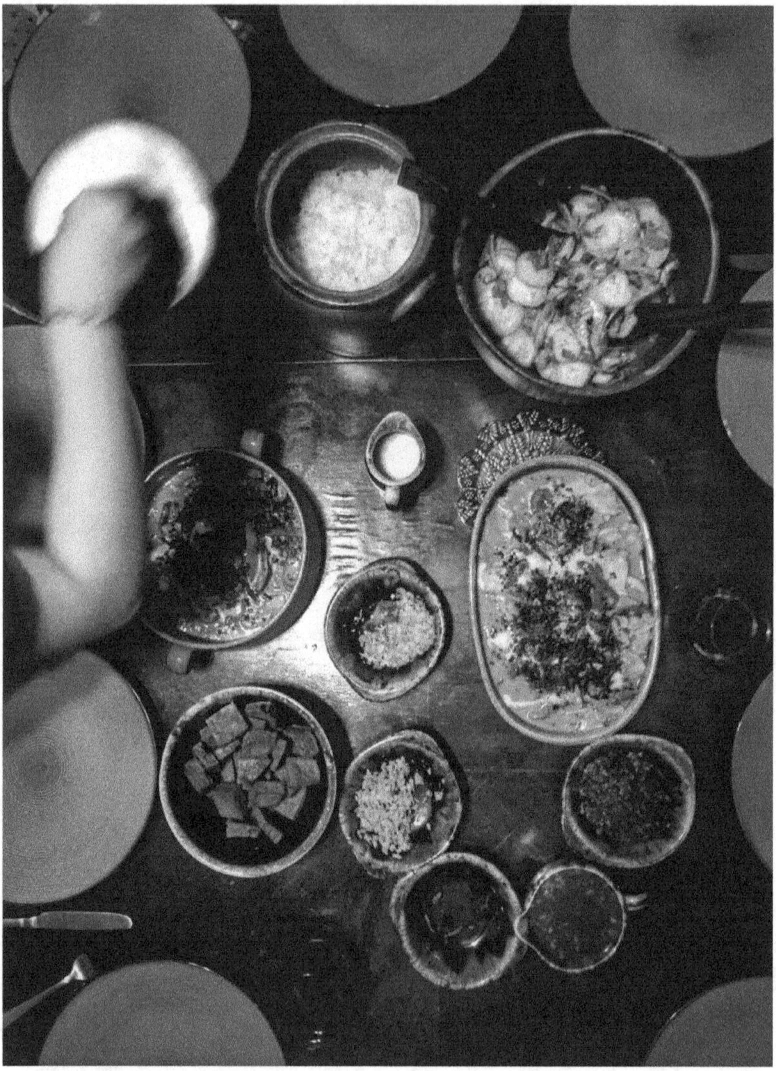

TABLE OF CONTENT

The information in the following pages is broadly considered a truthful and accurate account of facts and as such, any inattention, use, or misuse of the information in question by the reader will render any resulting actions solely under their purview. There are no scenarios in which the publisher or the original author of this work can be in any fashion deemed liable for any hardship or damages that may befall them after undertaking information described herein.

Additionally, the information in the following pages is intended only for informational purposes and should thus be thought of as universal. As befitting its nature, it is presented without assurance regarding its prolonged validity or interim quality. Trademarks that are mentioned are done without written consent and can in no way be considered an endorsement from the trademark holder.

Introduction

The Pegan Diet is a worldwide trending diet that owes its spread to its mysterious origin. Its true roots combine certain aspects of two diets - Paleo and Vegan, which don't add up well on paper. The term Pegan was coined by Dr. Mark Hyman, the director of the Cleveland Clinic Centre for Functional Medicine, who claims that the Pegan way of eating is not only the most sensible diet designed for the human race, but it is also the healthiest.

Pegan Diet includes about 50% of plant foods (fruits, vegetables and whole grains) that are low in calories but high in nutrition. The other 50% is rich in proteins from plants, healthy fats from nuts, seeds, fish and seafood and low-fat dairy products. In a word, Pegan Diet contains more nutrients rather than calories. Therefore, it will never make you obese or overweight because it has a low-calorie density (grams of calories per 100 grams).

Adopting Pegan Diet can help you to achieve an ideal weight without going through any kind of strict and hard dieting. This is because 1) Pegan Diet contains more fiber than any other diet. Fiber makes you feel full in addition fulfilled so that you don't need to take a large portion of food.

2) Pegan Diet contains various plant foods from which you can select the ones that will be favorable to you. For example, if you like apples and oranges but dislike broccoli, you can easily make a choice.

3) Pegan Diet is designed to help you burn more calories than any other diet. This is because it contains both kinds of nutrients: fats and carbohydrates. When your body burns the nutrients for energy, it will produce heat. The larger the number of nutrients, the more heat will be produced and in turn more calories will be burned.

Pegan Diet can provide your body with adequate nutrition for both brain and gut health.

The brains are made with 60% fats. Pegan Diet can improve your brain health in two ways:

(1) it contains a sufficient amount of omega 3 fatty acids, which are essential for the healthy function of the brain;

(2) it includes nuts, seeds, legumes and whole grains which are excellent sources of vegetable protein and healthy fats.

Pegan Diet can improve your memory power and brain function generally; enhance gut health to promote healthy digestion and break down of undigested food in the intestines; reduce skin inflammation in acne patients; protect against eczema by stopping the chain of inflammatory reactions in skin cells. How does it improve your gut health? Pegan Diet contains two kinds of fiber: soluble fiber (found in fruits, vegetables, nuts and legumes, especially oats) and insoluble fiber (found in whole grains). Soluble fiber helps reduce the risk of diverticulosis and diverticulitis. Insoluble fiber reduces constipation.

Pegan Diet can reduce the risk of inflammatory bowel disease by reducing intestinal permeability; improve bowel movements and treat diarrhea; help to prevent colon cancer.
Pegan Diet can promote gastric ulcer healing; decrease the incidence of gallstones; cure itchy skin conditions like atopic dermatitis (eczema), urticaria (hives) and psoriasis.

1. Sweet Potato Bisque

Preparation time: 15minutes

Cooking time: 45minutes

Servings: 4

Ingredients:

- 2 sweet potatoes, peeled and sliced
- 2 cups frozen butternut squash
- 2 (14.5-ounce) cans full-fat coconut milk
- 1 medium yellow onion, sliced
- 1 teaspoon minced garlic (2 cloves)
- 1 tablespoon dried basil
- 1 tablespoon chili powder
- 1 tablespoon ground cumin
- 1/2 cup water
- Pinch salt
- Freshly ground black pepper

Directions:

1. Combine the sweet potatoes, butternut squash, coconut milk, onion, garlic, dried basil, chili powder, cumin, and water in a slow cooker; mix well.

2. Cook on low heat.

3. Blend the soup until it's nice and creamy.

4. Season with salt and pepper.

Nutrition:

Calories: 447

Total fat: 8g

Protein: 72g

Sodium: 346

Fat: 19g

2. Chickpea Medley

Preparation time: 5minutes

Cooking time: 15minutes

Servings: 4

Ingredients:

- 2 tablespoons tahini
- 2 tablespoons coconut amines
- 1 (15-ounce) can chickpeas or 1.1/2 cups cooked chickpeas, rinsed and drained
- 1 cup finely chopped lightly packed spinach
- Carrot, peeled and grated

Directions:

1. Merge together the tahini and coconut amines in a bowl.
2. Add the chickpeas, spinach, and carrot to the bowl. Stir well and serve at room temperature.

3. Simple Swap: Coconut amines are almost like a sweeter, mellower version of soy sauce. However, if you want to use regular soy sauce or tamari, just use 11/2 tablespoons and add a dash of maple syrup or agave nectar to balance out the saltiness.

Nutrition:

Calories: 437

Total fat: 8g

Protein: 92g

Sodium: 246

Fat: 19g

3. Pasta with Lemon and Artichokes

Preparation time: 10minutes

Cooking time: 20minutes

Servings: 4

Ingredients:

- 16 ounces linguine or angel hair pasta
- 1/4 cup extra-virgin olive oil
- 8 garlic cloves, finely minced or pressed
- 2 (15-ounce) jars water-packed artichoke hearts, drained and quartered
- 2 tablespoons freshly squeezed lemon juice
- 1/4 cup thinly sliced fresh basil
- 1 teaspoon sea salt
- Freshly ground black pepper

Directions:

1. Use a large pot of water to a boil over high heat and cook the pasta until al dente according to the directions on the package.
2. While the pasta is cooking, heat the oil in a skillet over medium heat and cook the garlic, stirring often, for 1 to 2 minutes until it just begins to brown. Toss the garlic with the artichokes in a large bowl.
3. When the pasta is done, drain it and add it to the artichoke mixture, then add the lemon juice, basil, salt, and pepper. Gently stir and serve.

Nutrition:

Calories: 237

Total fat: 7g

Protein: 52g

Sodium: 346

Fat: 19g

4. Roasted Pine Nut Orzo

Preparation time: 10minutes

Cooking time: 15minutes

Servings: 3

Ingredients:

- 16 ounces orzo
- 1 cup diced roasted red peppers
- 1/4 cup pitted, chopped Klamath olives
- 4 garlic cloves, minced or pressed
- 3 tablespoons olive oil
- 1.1/2 tablespoons squeezed lemon juice
- 2 teaspoons balsamic vinegar
- 1 teaspoon sea salt
- 1/4 cup pine nuts
- 1/4 cup packed thinly sliced or torn fresh basil

Directions:

1. Use a large pot of water to a boil over medium-high heat and add the orzo. Cook, stirring often, for 10 minutes, or until the orzo has a chewy and firm texture. Drain well.

2. While the orzo is cooking, in a large bowl, combine the peppers, olives, garlic, olive oil, lemon juice, vinegar, and salt. Stir well.

3. In a dry skillet toasts the pine nuts over medium-low heat until aromatic and lightly browned, shaking the pan often so that they cook evenly

4. Upon reaching the desired texture and add it to the sauce mixture within a minute or so, to avoid clumping.

Nutrition:
Calories: 537
Total fat: 7g
Protein: 72g
Sodium: 246
Fat: 19g

5. Banana and Almond Butter Oats

Preparation Time: 10 minutes

Cooking time: 5 minutes

Servings: 2

Ingredients:

- 1 cup gluten-free moved oats
- 1 cup almond milk
- 1 cup of water
- 1 teaspoon cinnamon
- 2 tablespoons almond spread
- 1 banana, cut

Directions:

1. Mix the water and almond milk to a bubble in a little pot. Add the oats and diminish to a stew.
2. Cook until oats have consumed all fluid. Blend in cinnamon. Top with almond spread and banana and serve.

Nutrition:

Calories: 112;

Fat: 10g;

Protein: 9g;

Carbohydrates: 54g;

Fiber: 15g;

Sugar: 5g;

Sodium: 180mg

6. Red Tofu Curry

Preparation time: 15 minutes

Cooking time: 65 minutes

Servings: 4

Ingredients:

- 1 1/2 tablespoon canola oil
- 1 package extra-firm tofu
- 3 cups baby carrots
- 2 cups peeled red
- 2 onions,
- 3 teaspoons garlic
- 1 piece ginger
- 1.1/2 cups water
- 1 cup canned unsweetened coconut milk
- 1.1/2 tablespoons red curry paste
- 1 vegetable bouillon cube
- 1/2 teaspoon salt

- Cooked rice, for serving
- Fresh cilantro, for garnish

Directions:

1. Heat the oil in a skillet. Place the tofu and brown.
2. Merge all the ingredients and mix well.
3. Cook on low heat
4. Present over rice and garnished with cilantro.

Nutrition:

Calories: 617

Total fat: 2g

Protein: 32g

Sodium: 563mg

Fiber: 10g

7. Spicy Tomato-Lentil Stew

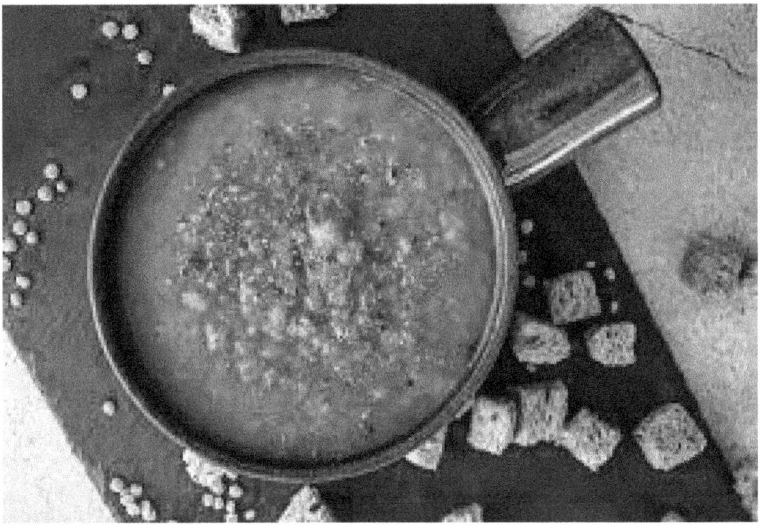

Preparation time: 15 minutes

Cooking time: 60 minutes

Servings: 5

Ingredients:

- 2 cups dry brown
- 1 can crushed tomatoes
- 1 can diced tomatoes
- 2 cups peeled potatoes

- 1 yellow onion
- 1/2 cup carrot
- 1/2 cup celery
- 2 tablespoons hot sauce
- 2 teaspoons garlic
- 2 teaspoons cumin
- 1 teaspoon chili
- 1/2 teaspoon coriander
- 1/4 teaspoon paprika
- 1 1/4 bay leaf
- pepper
- 4 bouillon cubes

Directions:

1. Merge all the ingredients and mix well.

2. Cook on low heat

3. Ready to serve.

Nutrition:

Calories: 517

Total fat: 2g

Protein: 32g

Sodium: 1,063mg

Fiber: 38g

8. Mixed-Bean Chili

Preparation time: 10minutes

Cooking time: 60 minutes

Servings: 4

Ingredients:

- 5 (15-ounce) cans your choice beans, drained and rinsed
- 1 (15-ounce) can diced tomatoes, with juice
- 1 (6-ounce) can tomato paste
- 1 cup water
- 1 green bell pepper, diced
- 2 cups stemmed and chopped kale
- 1/2 medium yellow onion, diced
- 2 tablespoons ground cumin
- 1 tablespoon chili powder
- 1 teaspoon minced garlic (2 cloves)
- 1 teaspoon cayenne pepper

- Pinch salt

Directions:

1. Place the beans, diced tomatoes, tomato paste, water, bell pepper, kale, onion, cumin, chili powder, garlic, and cayenne pepper in a slow cooker.
2. Season with salt and serve.

Nutrition:

Calories: 417

Total fat: 2g

Protein: 72g

Sodium: 463mg

Fiber: 10g

9. Butternut Squash Soup

Preparation time: 10minutes

Cooking time: 70 minutes

Servings: 4

Ingredients:

- 2 (10-ounce) packages frozen butternut squash
- 6 cups water
- 1 medium yellow onion, chopped
- 1 teaspoon minced garlic (2 cloves)
- 5 vegetable bouillon cubes
- 2 bay leaves
- 1/4 teaspoon freshly ground black pepper
- 1/8 teaspoon cayenne pepper
- 1 (8-ounce) package vegan cream cheese, cut into chunks

Directions:

1. Combine the butternut squash, water, onion, garlic, bouillon cubes, bay leaves, black pepper, and cayenne pepper in a slow cooker. Stir to mix.
2. Cook on low heat.
3. Remove the bay leaves.
4. Purée half of the soup using a blender.
5. Stir in the cream cheese. Cover and cook on low for 30 minutes longer.

Nutrition:

Calories: 617

Total fat: 2g

Protein: 82g

Sodium: 563mg

Fiber: 10g

10. Split-Pea Soup

Preparation time: 10minutes

Cooking time: 65 minutes

Servings: 5

Ingredients:

- 1-pound dried green split peas, rinsed
- 6 cups water
- 3 carrots, diced
- 3 celery stalks, diced
- 1 medium russet potato, peeled and diced
- 1 small yellow onion, diced
- 1.1/2 teaspoons minced garlic (3 cloves)
- 5 vegetable bouillon cubes
- 1 bay leaf
- Freshly ground black pepper

Directions:

1. Combine the split peas, water, carrots, celery, potato, onion, garlic, bouillon cubes, and bay leaf in a slow cooker; mix well.
2. Cook on low heat, and season with pepper.

Nutrition:

Calories: 817

Total fat: 2g

Protein: 82g

Sodium: 363mg

Fiber: 10g

11. Tomato Bisque

Preparation time: 10minutes

Cooking time: 65 minutes

Servings: 4

Ingredients:

- 2 (28-ounce) cans crushed tomatoes
- 1 (28-ounce) can whole peeled tomatoes, with juice
- 1 (15-ounce) can white beans, drained and rinsed
- 1/2 cup cashew pieces
- 2 vegetable bouillon cubes
- 1 tablespoon dried basil
- 2 teaspoons minced garlic (4 cloves)
- 3 cups water
- Pinch salt
- Freshly ground black pepper

Directions:

1. Combine the crushed tomatoes, whole peeled tomatoes, white beans, cashew pieces, bouillon cubes, dried basil, garlic, and water in a slow cooker.
2. Cook on low heat.
3. Blend the soup until smooth. Season with salt and pepper.

Nutrition:

Calories: 817

Total fat: 2g

Protein: 82g

Sodium:

12. Cheesy Potato-Broccoli Soup

Preparation time: 15minutes

Cooking time: 70minutes

Servings: 4

Ingredients:

- 2 pounds red or Yukon potatoes, chopped
- 1 (10-ounce) bag frozen broccoli
- 2 cups unsweetened nondairy milk
- 1 small yellow onion, chopped
- 1.1/2 teaspoons minced garlic (3 cloves)
- 3 vegetable bouillon cubes
- 4 cups water
- 1 cup melts able vegan Cheddar-cheese shreds (such as Diana or Follow Your Heart)
- Pinch salt
- Freshly ground black pepper

Directions:

1. Combine the potatoes, broccoli, nondairy milk, onion, garlic, bouillon cubes, and water in a slow cooker; mix well.
2. Cook on low heat.
3. Forty-five minutes before serving, use an immersion blender (or a regular blender, working in batches) to blend the soup until it's nice and creamy.
4. Stir in the vegan cheese, cover, and cook for another 45 minutes.
5. Season with salt and pepper.

Nutrition:

Calories: 517

Total fat: 2g

Protein: 92g

Sodium:

13. Vegetable Stew

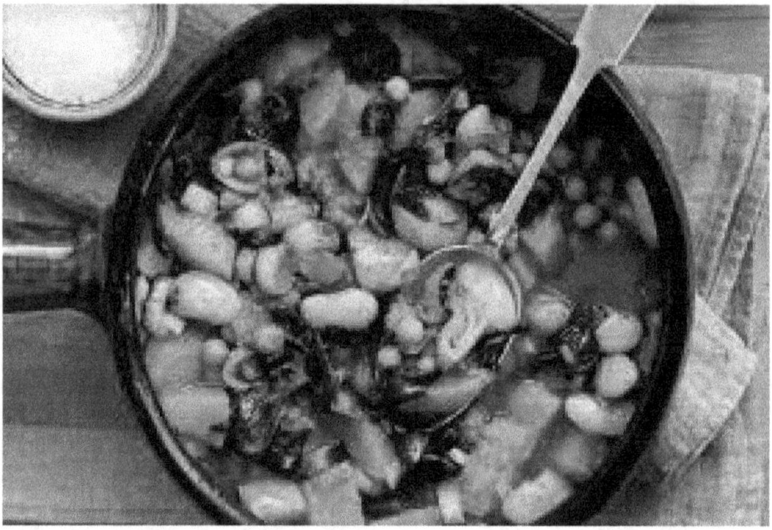

Preparation time: 15minutes

Cooking time: 65minutes

Servings: 4

Ingredients:

- 1 (28-ounce) can diced tomatoes, with juice
- 1 can white beans
- 1 cup diced green beans

- 2 medium potatoes, diced
- 1 cup frozen carrots and peas mix
- 1 small yellow onion, diced
- 1 (1-inch) piece ginger, peeled and minced
- 1 teaspoon minced garlic (2 cloves)
- 3 cups Vegetable Broth
- 2 teaspoons ground cumin
- 1/2 teaspoon red pepper flakes
- Juice of 1/2 lemon
- 1 cup dried pasta
- Pinch salt
- Freshly ground black pepper
- Pesto, for serving

Directions:

1. Combine the diced tomatoes, white beans, green beans, potatoes, carrots and peas mix, onion,

ginger, garlic, vegetable broth, cumin, red pepper flakes, and lemon juice in a slow cooker.

2. Cook on low heat.
3. Pour with salt and pepper and serve with a dollop of pesto.

Nutrition:

Calories: 617

Total fat: 2g

Protein: 92g

Sodium: 356

Fat: 16g

14. Frijoles De La Olla

Preparation time: 15minutes

Cooking time: 65minutes

Servings: 4

Ingredients:

- 1-pound dry pinto beans, rinsed
- 1 small yellow onion, diced
- 1 jalapeño pepper, seeded and finely chopped
- 1.1/2 teaspoons minced garlic (3 cloves)
- 1 tablespoon ground cumin
- 1/2 teaspoon Mexican oregano (optional)
- 1 teaspoon red pepper flakes (optional)
- 4 cups water
- 2 tablespoons salt

Directions:

1. Place the beans, onion, jalapeño, garlic, cumin, oregano (if using), red pepper flakes (if using), water, and salt in a slow cooker.
2. Cook on low heat.

Nutrition

Total fat: 2g

Protein: 82g

Sodium: 346

Fat: 16g

15. Vegetable Hominy Soup

Preparation time: 15minutes

Cooking time: 30minutes

Servings: 4

Ingredients:

- 1 (28-ounce) can hominy, drained
- 1 (28-ounce) can diced tomatoes with green chills
- 5 medium red or Yukon potatoes, diced
- 1 large yellow onion, diced
- 2 cups chopped carrots
- 2 celery stalks, chopped
- 2 teaspoons minced garlic (4 cloves)
- 2 tablespoons chopped cilantro
- 1.1/2 tablespoons ground cumin
- 1.1/2 tablespoons seasoned salt
- 1 tablespoon chili powder
- 1 bay leaf

- 4 vegetable bouillon cubes
- 5 cups water
- Pinch salt
- Freshly ground black pepper

Directions:

1. Combine the hominy, diced tomatoes, potatoes, onion, carrots, celery, garlic, cilantro, cumin, seasoned salt, chili powder, bay leaf, vegetable bouillon, and water in a slow cooker; mix well. Cook on low heat.
2. . Remove the bay leaf. Season with salt and pepper.

Nutrition:

Calories: 417

Total fat: 2g

Protein: 72g

Sodium: 346

Fat: 16g

16. Lentil-Quinoa Chili

Preparation time: 15minutes

Cooking time: 30minutes

Servings: 4

Ingredients:

- 1/2 cup dry green lentils
- 1 can black beans
- 1/3 cup uncooked quinoa, rinsed
- 1 small yellow onion, diced
- 2 medium carrots, diced
- 2 teaspoons ground cumin
- 2 teaspoons chili powder
- 1.1/2 teaspoons minced garlic (3 cloves)
- 1 teaspoon dried oregano
- 3 vegetable bouillon cubes
- 1 bay leaf
- 4 cups water

- Pinch salt

Directions:

1. Place the lentils, black beans, quinoa, onion, carrots, cumin, chili powder, garlic, oregano, bouillon cubes, bay leaf, and water in a slow cooker; mix well.
2. Cook on low heat.
3. Remove the bay leaf, season with salt, and serve.

Nutrition:

Calories: 617

Total fat: 2g

Protein: 72g

Sodium: 346

Fat: 16g

17. Eggplant Curry

Preparation time: 15minutes

Cooking time: 35minutes

Servings: 5

Ingredients:

- 5 cups chopped eggplant
- 4 cups chopped zucchini
- 2 cups stemmed and chopped kale
- 1 (15-ounce) can full-fat coconut milk
- 1 (14.5-ounce) can diced tomatoes, drained
- 1 (6-ounce) can tomato paste
- 1 medium yellow onion, chopped
- 2 teaspoons minced garlic (4 cloves)
- 1 tablespoon curry powder
- 1 tablespoon gram masala
- 1/4 teaspoon cayenne pepper
- 1/4 teaspoon ground cumin

- 1 teaspoon salt
- Cooked rice, for serving

Directions:

1. Combine the eggplant, zucchini, kale, coconut milk, diced tomatoes, tomato paste, onion, garlic, curry powder, gram masala, cayenne pepper, cumin, and salt in a slow cooker; mix well.
2. Cook on low heat.

Nutrition:

Calories: 417

Total fat: 2g

Protein: 72g

Sodium: 346

Fat: 19g

18. Meaty Chili

Preparation time: 15minutes

Cooking time: 40minutes

Servings: 5

Ingredients:

- 1 tablespoon olive oil
- 2 packages of faux-ground-beef veggie crumble (such as Beyond Meat)
- 1 large red onion, chopped
- 1 large jalapeño pepper, seeded and chopped
- 2 1/2 teaspoons minced garlic
- 1 can diced tomatoes
- 1 can kidney beans
- 1 can black beans
- 1/2 cup frozen corn
- 1/4 cup chili powder
- 2 tablespoons ground cumin

- 1 teaspoon smoked paprika
- 1 vegetable bouillon cube
- 1.1/2 cups water

Directions:

1. Heat the olive oil in a sauté pan over medium-high heat. Add the veggie crumbles, onion, jalapeño, and garlic, and cook for 3 to 4 minutes, stirring occasionally.
2. Combine the veggie-crumble mixture, diced tomatoes, kidney beans, black beans, frozen corn, chili powder, cumin, smoked paprika, bouillon cube, and water in a slow cooker; mix well.
3. Cook on low heat.

Nutrition:

Calories: 547

Total fat: 8g

Protein: 62g

Sodium: 346

Fat: 19g

19. Black Bean Burgers

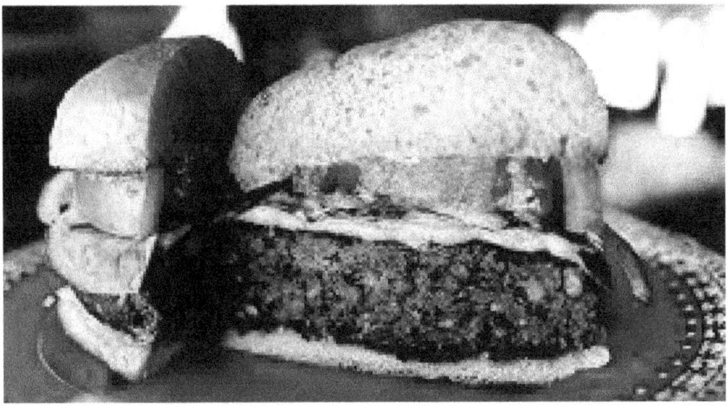

Preparation Time: 5 Minutes

Cooking Time: 20 Minutes

Servings: 4

Ingredients:

- 1 onion, diced
- 1/2 cup corn nibs
- 2 cloves garlic, minced
- 1/2 teaspoon oregano, dried
- 1/2 cup flour

- 1 jalapeno pepper, small
- 2 cups black beans, mashed & canned
- 1/4 cup breadcrumbs (vegan)
- 2 teaspoons parsley, minced
- 1/4 teaspoon cumin
- 1 tablespoon olive oil
- 2 teaspoons chili powder
- 1/2 red pepper, diced
- Sea salt to taste

Directions:

1. Set your flour on a plate, and then get out your garlic, onion, peppers and oregano, throwing it in a pan.
2. Cook over medium-high heat, and then cook until the onions are translucent.

3. Place the peppers in, and sauté until tender.
4. Cook for two minutes, and then set it to the side.
5. Use a potato masher to mash your black beans, and then stir in the vegetables, cumin, breadcrumbs, parsley, salt and chili powder, and then divide it into six patties.
6. Coat each side, and then cook until it's fried on each side.

Nutrition:

Calories: 211

Carbs: 12g

Fat: 7g

Protein: 12g

20. Dijon Maple Burgers

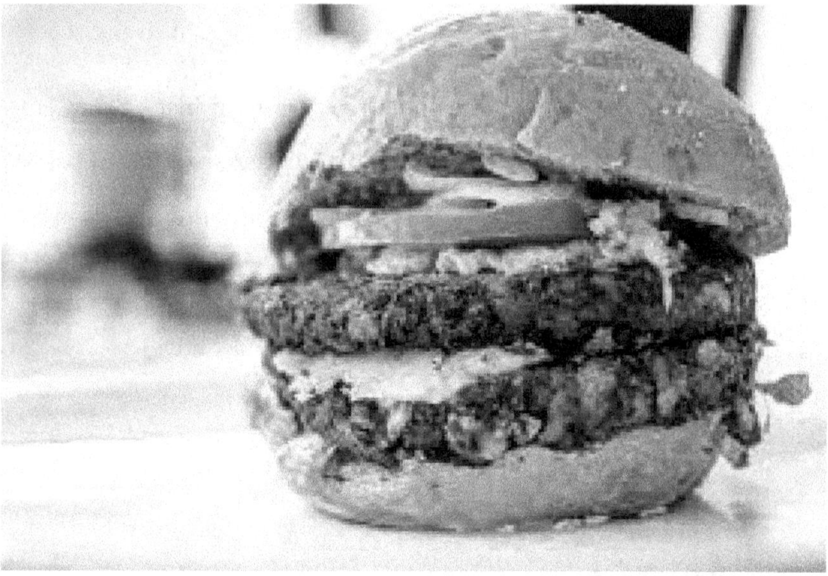

Preparation Time: 10 Minutes

Cooking Time: 40 Minutes

Servings: 12

Ingredients:

- 1 red bell pepper
- 19 ounces can chickpeas, rinsed & drained
- 1 cup almonds, ground

- 2 teaspoons Dijon mustard
- 1 teaspoon oregano
- 1/2 teaspoon sage
- 1 cup spinach, fresh
- 1 – 1/2 cups rolled oats
- 1 clove garlic, pressed
- 1/2 lemon, juiced
- 2 teaspoons maple syrup, pure

Directions:

1. Get out a baking sheet. Line it with parchment paper.
2. Cut your red pepper in half and then take the seeds out. Place it on your baking sheet, and roast in the oven while you prepare your other Ingredients:

3. Process your chickpeas, almonds, mustard and maple syrup together in a food processor.
4. Add in your lemon juice, oregano, sage, garlic and spinach, processing again. Make sure it's combined, but don't puree it.
5. Once your red bell pepper is softened, which should roughly take ten minutes, add this to the processor as well. Add in your oats, mixing well.

Nutrition:

Calories: 209

Carbs: 11g

Fat: 5g

Protein: 9g

21. Hearty Black Lentil Curry

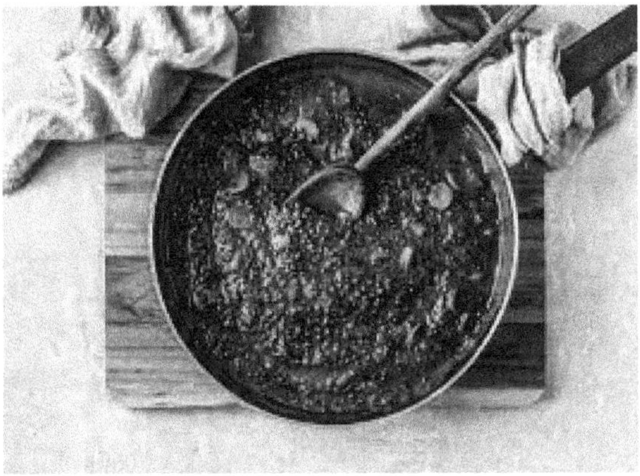

Preparation Time: 15 Minutes

Cooking Time: 6 Hours

Servings: 7

Ingredients:

- 1 cup of black lentils, rinsed and soaked overnight
- 14 ounces of chopped tomatoes
- 2 large white onions, peeled and sliced
- 1 1/2 teaspoon of minced garlic
- 1 teaspoon of grated ginger

- 1 red chili
- 1 teaspoon of salt
- 1/4 teaspoon of red chili powder
- 1 teaspoon of paprika
- 1 teaspoon of ground turmeric
- 2 teaspoons of ground cumin
- 2 teaspoons of ground coriander
- 1/2 cup of chopped coriander
- 4-ounce of vegetarian butter
- 1 fluid of ounce water
- 2 fluid of ounce vegetarian double cream

Directions:

1. Place a large pan over a moderate heat, add butter and let heat until melt.

2. Add the onion and garlic and ginger and let cook for 10 to 15 minutes or until onions are caramelized.
3. Then stir in salt, red chili powder, paprika, turmeric, cumin, ground coriander, and water.
4. Transfer this mixture to a 6-quarts slow cooker and add tomatoes and red chili.
5. Drain lentils, add to slow cooker and stir until just mix.
6. Plug in slow cooker; adjust cooking time to 6 hours and let cook on low heat setting.
7. When the lentils are done, stir in cream and adjust the seasoning.
8. Serve with boiled rice or whole wheat bread.

Nutrition:
Calories: 171
Carbs: 10g
Fat: 7g
Protein: 12g

22. Flavorful Refried Beans

Preparation Time: 15 Minutes

Cooking Time: 8 Hours

Servings: 8

Ingredients:

- 3 cups of pinto beans, rinsed
- 1 small jalapeno pepper, seeded and chopped
- 1 medium-sized white onion, peeled and sliced
- 2 tablespoons of minced garlic
- 5 teaspoons of salt
- 2 teaspoons of ground black pepper
- 1/4 teaspoon of ground cumin
- 9 cups of water

Directions:

1. Using a 6-quarts slow cooker, place all the Ingredients: and stir until it mixes properly.

2. Cover the top, plug in the slow cooker; adjust the cooking time to 6 hours, let it cook on high heat setting and add more water if the beans get too dry.
3. When the beans are done, drain them and reserve the liquid.
4. Mash the beans using a potato masher and pour in the reserved cooking liquid until it reaches your desired mixture.
5. Serve immediately.

Nutrition:

Calories: 198

Carbs: 22g

Fat: 7g

Protein: 19g

23. Smoky Red Beans and Rice

Preparation Time: 15 Minutes

Cooking Time: 5 Hours

Servings: 8

Ingredients:

- 30 ounces of cooked red beans
- 1 cup of brown rice, uncooked
- 1 cup of chopped green pepper
- 1 cup of chopped celery
- 1 cup of chopped white onion
- 1 1/2 teaspoon of minced garlic
- 1/2 teaspoon of salt
- 1/4 teaspoon of cayenne pepper
- 1 teaspoon of smoked paprika
- 2 teaspoons of dried thyme
- 1 bay leaf

- 2 1/3 cups of vegetable broth

Directions:

1. Using a 6-quarts slow cooker, all the Ingredients are except for the rice, salt, and cayenne pepper.
2. Stir until it mixes appropriately and then cover the top.
3. Plug in the slow cooker; adjust the cooking time to 4 hours, and steam on a low heat setting.
4. Then pour in and stir the rice, salt, cayenne pepper and continue cooking for an additional 2 hours at a high heat setting.

Nutrition:

Calories: 234

Carbs: 13g

Fat: 7g

Protein: 19g

24. Spicy Black-Eyed Peas

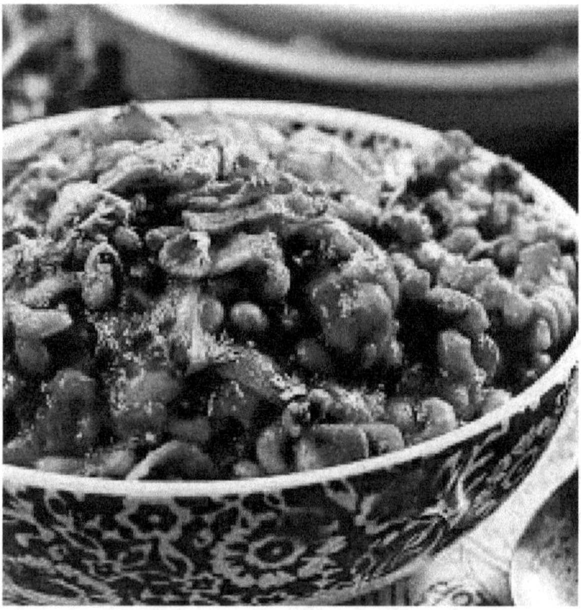

Preparation Time: 15 Minutes

Cooking Time: 60 Minutes

Servings: 8

Ingredients:

- 32-ounce black-eyed peas, uncooked
- 1 cup of chopped orange bell pepper

- 1 cup of chopped celery
- 8-ounce of chipotle peppers, chopped
- 1 cup of chopped carrot
- 1 cup of chopped white onion
- 1 teaspoon of minced garlic
- 3/4 teaspoon of salt
- 1/2 teaspoon of ground black pepper
- 2 teaspoons of liquid smoke flavoring
- 2 teaspoons of ground cumin
- 1 tablespoon of adobo sauce
- 2 tablespoons of olive oil
- 1 tablespoon of apple cider vinegar
- 4 cups of vegetable broth

Directions:

1. Place a medium-sized non-stick skillet pan over an average temperature of heat; add the bell peppers, carrot, onion, garlic, oil and vinegar.

2. Stir until it mixes properly and let it cook for 5 to 8 minutes or until it gets translucent.

3. Transfer this mixture to a 6-quarts slow cooker and add the peas, chipotle pepper, adobo sauce and the vegetable broth.

4. Stir until mixes properly and cover the top.

5. Plug in the slow cooker; adjust the cooking time to 8 hours and let it cook on the low heat setting or until peas are soft.

Nutrition:

Calories: 211

Carbs: 22g

Fat: 7g

Protein: 19g

25. Creamy Artichoke Soup

Preparation Time: 5 Minutes

Cooking Time: 40 Minutes

Servings: 4

Ingredients:

- 1 can artichoke hearts, drained
- 3 cups vegetable broth
- 2 tablespoon lemon juice
- 1 small onion, finely cut
- 2 cloves garlic, crushed
- 3 tablespoons olive oil
- 2 tablespoon flour
- 1/2 cup vegan cream

Directions:

1. Gently sauté the onion and garlic in some olive oil.

2. Add the flour, whisking constantly, and then add the hot vegetable broth slowly, while still whisking. Cook for about 5 minutes.
3. Blend the artichoke, lemon juice, salt and pepper until smooth. Add the puree to the broth mix, stir well, and then stir in the cream.
4. Cook until heated through. Garnish with a swirl of vegan cream or a sliver of artichoke.

Nutrition:

Calories: 211

Carbs: 12g

Fat: 7g

Protein: 11g

26. Super Rad-ish Avocado Salad

Preparation Time: 10 Minutes

Cooking Time: 25 Minutes

Servings: 2

Ingredients:

- 6 shredded carrots
- 6 ounces diced radishes
- 1 diced avocado
- 1/3 cup ponzu

Directions:

1. Bring all the above ingredients together in a serving bowl and toss.
2. Enjoy!

Nutrition:

Calories: 211

Carbs: 9g

Fat: 7g

Protein: 12g

27. Beauty School Ginger Cucumbers

Preparation Time: 10 Minutes

Cooking Time: 5 Minutes

Servings: 2

Ingredients:

- 1 sliced cucumber
- 3 teaspoon rice wine vinegar
- 1 1/2 tablespoon sugar
- 1 teaspoon minced ginger

Directions:

1. Bring all of the above ingredients together in a mixing bowl, and toss the ingredients well.
2. Enjoy!

Nutrition:

Calories: 210

Carbs: 14g

Fat: 7g

Protein: 19g

28. Mushroom Salad

Preparation Time: 10 Minutes

Cooking Time: 20 Minutes

Servings: 2

Ingredients:

- 1 tablespoon butter
- 1/2-pound cremini mushrooms, chopped
- 2 tablespoons extra-virgin olive oil
- Salt and black pepper to taste
- 2 bunches arugula
- 4 slices prosciutto
- 1 tablespoon apple cider vinegar
- 4 sundried tomatoes in oil, drained and chopped
- Fresh parsley leaves, chopped

Directions:

1. Heat a pan with butter and half of the oil.

2. Add the mushrooms, salt, and pepper. Stir-fry for 3 minutes. Reduce heat. Stir again, and cook for 3 minutes more.
3. Add rest of the oil and vinegar. Stir and cook for 1 minute.
4. Place arugula on a platter, add prosciutto on top, add the mushroom mixture, sundried tomatoes, more salt and pepper, parsley, and serve.

Nutrition:

Calories: 191

Carbs: 6g

Fat: 7g

Protein: 17g

29. Red Quinoa and Black Bean Soup

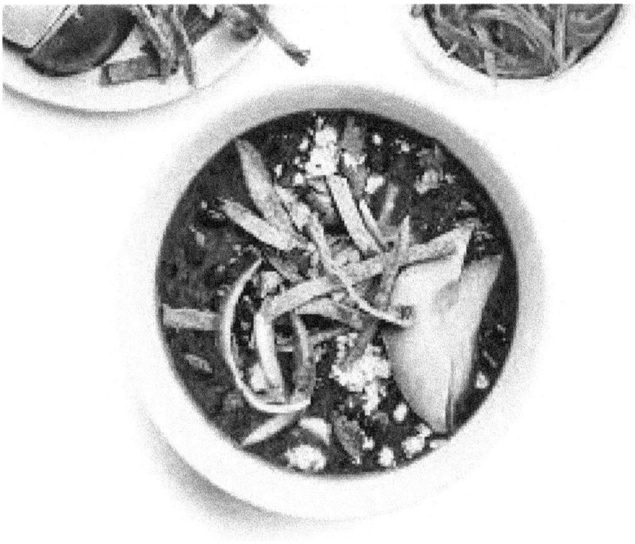

Preparation Time: 5 Minutes

Cooking Time: 40 Minutes

Servings: 6

Ingredients:

- 1/4 cup red quinoa
- 4 minced garlic cloves
- 1/2 tablespoon coconut oil

- 1 diced jalapeno
- 3 cups diced onion
- 2 teaspoon cumin
- 1 chopped sweet potato
- 1 teaspoon coriander
- 1 teaspoon chili powder
- 5 cups vegetable broth
- 15 ounces' black beans
- 1/2 teaspoon cayenne pepper
- 2 cups spinach

Directions:

1. Begin by bringing the quinoa into a saucepan to boil with two cups of water. Allow the quinoa to simmer for twenty minutes. Next, remove the quinoa from the heat.

2. To the side, heat the oil, the onion, and the garlic together in a large soup pot.
3. Add the jalapeno and the sweet potato and sauté for an additional seven minutes.
4. Next, add all the spices and the broth and bring the soup to a simmer for twenty-five minutes. The potatoes should be soft.
5. Before serving, add the quinoa, the black beans, and the spinach to the mix. Season, and serve warm. Enjoy.

Nutrition:

Calories: 211

Carbs: 22g

Fat: 7g

Protein: 19g

30. October Potato Soup

Preparation Time: 5 Minutes

Cooking Time: 20 Minutes

Servings: 3

Ingredients:

- 4 minced garlic cloves
- 2 teaspoon coconut oil
- 3 diced celery stalks
- 1 diced onion
- 2 teaspoon yellow mustard seeds
- 5 diced Yukon potatoes
- 6 cups vegetable broth
- 1 teaspoon oregano
- 1 teaspoon paprika
- 1/2 teaspoon cayenne pepper
- 1 teaspoon chili powder

- Salt and pepper to taste

Directions:

1. Begin by sautéing the garlic and the mustard seeds together in the oil in a large soup pot.
2. Next, add the onion and sauté the mixture for another five minutes.
3. Add the celery, the broth, the potatoes, and all the spices, and continue to stir.
4. Allow the soup to simmer for thirty minutes without a cover.
5. Next, Position about three cups of the soup in a blender, and puree the soup until you've reached a smooth consistency. Pour this back into the big soup pot, stir, and serve warm. Enjoy.

Nutrition:

Calories: 203

Carbs: 12g

Fat: 7g

Protein: 9g

31. Rice with Asparagus and Cauliflower

Preparation Time: 5 Minutes

Cooking Time: 20 Minutes

Servings: 2

Ingredients:

- 3 ounces' asparagus
- 3 ounces' cauliflower, chopped
- 2 ounces' tomato sauce
- 1/2 cup of brown rice
- 3/4 cup of water
- 1/3 teaspoon salt
- 1/4 teaspoon ground black pepper
- 1/4 teaspoon garlic powder
- 1 tablespoon olive oil

Directions:

1. Take a medium saucepan, place it over medium heat, add oil, add asparagus and cauliflower and then sauté for 5 to 7 minutes until golden brown.
2. Season with garlic powder, salt, and black pepper, stir in tomato sauce, and then cook for 1 minute.
3. Add rice, pour in water, stir until mixed, cover with a lid and cook for 10 to 12 minutes until rice has absorbed all the liquid and become tender.
4. When done, remove the pan from heat, fluff rice with a fork, and then serve.

Nutrition:

Calories: 257

Carbs: 4g

Fat: 4g

Protein: 40g

32. Spaghetti with Tomato Sauce

Preparation Time: 5 Minutes

Cooking Time: 15 Minutes

Servings: 2

Ingredients:

- 4 ounces' spaghetti
- 2 green onions, greens, and whites separated
- 1/8 teaspoon coconut sugar
- 3 ounces' tomato sauce
- 1 tablespoon olive oil
- 1/3 teaspoon salt
- 1/4 teaspoon ground black pepper

Directions:

1. Prepare the spaghetti, and for this, cook it according to the Directions on the packet and then set aside.

2. Then take a skillet pan, place it over medium heat, add oil and when hot, add white parts of green onions and cook for 2 minutes until tender.
3. Add tomato sauce, season with salt and black pepper and bring it to a boil.
4. Switch heat to medium-low level, simmer sauce for 1 minute, then add the cooked spaghetti and toss until mixed.
5. Divide spaghetti between two plates, and then serve.

Nutrition:

Calories: 265

Carbs: 8g

Fat: 2g

Protein: 7g

33. Crispy Cauliflower

Preparation Time: 5 Minutes

Cooking Time: 15 Minutes

Servings: 2

Ingredients:

- 6 ounces of cauliflower florets
- 1/2 of zucchini, sliced
- 1/2 teaspoon of sea salt
- 1/2 tablespoon curry powder
- 1/4 teaspoon maple syrup
- 2 tablespoons olive oil

Directions:

1. Switch on the oven, then set it to 450 degrees F and let it preheat.
2. Meanwhile, take a medium bowl, add cauliflower florets and zucchini slices, add remaining

ingredients reserving 1 tablespoon oil, and toss until well coated.

3. Take a medium skillet pan, place it over medium-high heat, add remaining oil and wait until it gets hot.

4. Spread cauliflower and zucchini in a single layer and sauté for 5 minutes, tossing frequently.

5. Then transfer the pan into the oven and then bake for 8 to 10 minutes until vegetables have turned golden brown and thoroughly cooked, stirring halfway.

Nutrition:

Calories: 161

Carbs: 2g

Fat: 2g

Protein: 7g

34. Avocado Toast with Chickpeas

Preparation Time: 5 Minutes

Cooking Time: 5 Minutes

Servings: 2

Ingredients:

- 1/2 of avocado, peeled, pitted
- 4 tablespoons canned chickpeas, liquid reserved
- 1 tablespoon lime juice
- 1 teaspoon apple cider vinegar
- 2 slices of bread, toasted
- 1/4 teaspoon salt
- 1/4 teaspoon paprika
- 1 teaspoon olive oil

Directions:

1. Take a medium skillet pan, place it over medium heat, add oil and when hot, add chickpeas and cook for 2 minutes.

2. Sprinkle 1/8 teaspoon each salt and paprika over chickpeas, toss to coat, and then remove the pan from heat.
3. Place avocado in a bowl, mash by using a fork, drizzle with lime juice and vinegar and stir until well mixed.
4. Spread mashed avocado over bread slices, scatter chickpeas on top and then serve.

Nutrition:

Calories: 235

Carbs: 5g

Fat: 5g

Protein: 31g

35. Green Onion Soup

Preparation Time: 5 Minutes

Cooking Time: 12 Minutes

Servings: 2

Ingredients:

- 6 green onions, chopped
- 7 ounces diced potatoes
- 1/3 teaspoon salt
- 2 tablespoons olive oil
- 1/4 cup vegetable broth
- 1/4 teaspoon ground white pepper
- 1/4 teaspoon ground coriander

Directions:

1. Take a small pan, place potato in it, cover with water, and then place the pan over medium heat.

2. Boil the potato until cooked and tender, and when done, drain the potatoes and set aside until required.
3. Return saucepan over low heat, add oil and add green onions and cook for 5 minutes until cooked.
4. Season with salt, pepper, and coriander, add potatoes, pour in vegetable broth, stir until mixed and bring it to simmer.
5. Then remove the pan from heat and blend the mixture by using an immersion blender until creamy.
6. Taste to adjust seasoning, then ladle soup into bowls and then serve.

Nutrition:

Calories: 191

Carbs: 1g

Fat: 1g

Protein: 15g

36. Potato Soup

Preparation Time: 5 Minutes

Cooking Time: 12 Minutes

Servings: 2

Ingredients:

- 2 potatoes, peeled, cubed
- 1/3 teaspoon salt
- 1/2 cup vegetable broth
- 3/4 cup of water
- 1/8 teaspoon ground black pepper
- 1 tablespoon Cajun seasoning

Directions:

1. Take a small pan, place potato cubes in it, cover with water and vegetable broth, and then place the pan over medium heat.
2. Boil the potato until cooked and tender, and when done, remove the pan from heat and blend the

mixture by using an immersion blender until creamy.

3. Return pan over medium-low heat, add remaining Ingredients: stir until mixed and bring it to a simmer.
4. Taste to adjust seasoning, then ladle soup into bowls and then serve.

Nutrition:

Calories: 203

Carbs: 5g

Fat: 6g

Protein: 37g

37. Teriyaki Eggplant

Preparation Time: 5 Minutes

Cooking Time: 15 Minutes

Servings: 2

Ingredients:

- 1/2-pound eggplant
- 1 green onion, chopped
- 1/2 teaspoon grated ginger
- 1/2 teaspoon minced garlic
- 1/3 cup soy sauce
- 1 tablespoon coconut sugar
- 1/2 tablespoon apple cider vinegar
- 1 tablespoon olive oil

Directions:

1. Prepare vegan teriyaki sauce and for this, take a medium bowl, add ginger, garlic, soy sauce, vinegar,

and sugar in it and then whisk until sugar has dissolved completely.

2. Cut eggplant into cubes, add them into vegan teriyaki sauce, toss until well coated and marinate for 10 minutes.
3. When ready to cook, take a grill pan, place it over medium-high heat, grease it with oil, and when hot, add marinated eggplant.
4. Cook for 3 to 4 minutes per side until nicely browned and beginning to charred, drizzling with excess marinade frequently and transfer to a plate.
5. Sprinkle green onion on top of the eggplant and then serve.

Nutrition:

Calories: 132

Carbs: 4g

Fat: 4g

Protein: 13g

38. Broccoli Stir-Fry with Sesame Seeds

Preparation Time: 10 Minutes

Cooking Time: 8 Minutes

Servings: 4

Ingredients:

- Two tablespoons extra-virgin olive oil (optional)
- One tablespoon grated fresh ginger
- cups broccoli florets
- ¼teaspoon sea salt (optional)
- Two garlic cloves, minced
- Two tablespoons toasted sesame seeds

Directions:

1. Heat the olive oil (if desired) in a large nonstick skillet over medium-high heat until shimmering.
2. Fold in the ginger, broccoli, and sea salt (if desired) and stir-fry for 5 to 7 minutes, or until the broccoli is browned.

3. Cook the garlic until tender, about 30 seconds.

4. Sprinkle with the sesame seeds and serve warm.

Nutrition:

Calories: 135

Fat: 10.9g

Carbs: 9.7g

Protein: 4.1g

Fiber: 3.3g

39. Bream

Preparation time: 10minutes

Cooking time: 60minutes

Servings: 4

Ingredients:

- Olive oil cooking spray
- 2 medium zucchinis, cut into 1/2inch-thick rounds
- 2 gold potatoes, thinly sliced
- 4 tomatoes, sliced
- 1.3/4 cups tomato sauce
- 10 garlic cloves cut into large chunks
- 1.1/2 tablespoons olive oil
- 4 teaspoons dried basil
- 2 teaspoons dried oregano
- Teaspoon sea salt

Directions:

1. In a large bowl, combine the zucchini, potatoes, tomatoes, tomato sauce, garlic, olive oil, basil, oregano, and salt and stir well. Pour the vegetable into the dish.
2. Bake for 30 minutes, stir well, and bake for another 30 minutes, or until the potatoes are tender. Stir again and serve.

Nutrition:

Calories: 337

Total fat: 8

Protein: 82g

Sodium: 346

Fat: 19g

40. Green-Glory Soup (Pressure- Pot)

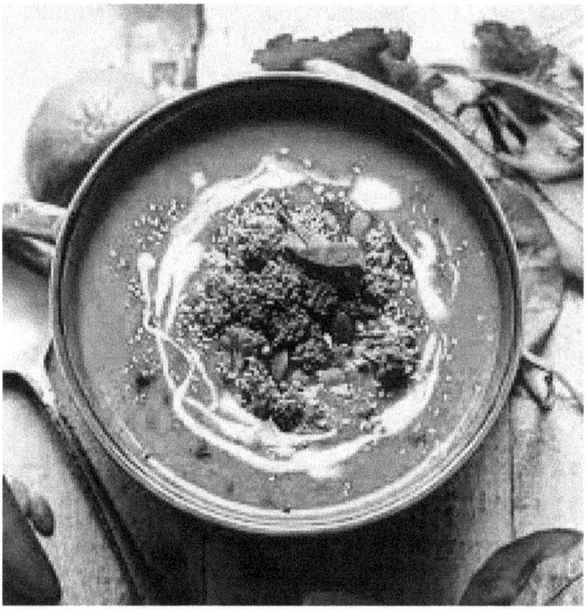

Preparation time: 10 minutes

Cooking time: 15 minutes

Servings: 4

Ingredients:

- 1 head cauliflower (florets)
- 1 onion (diced)

- 2 cloves garlic (minced)
- 1 cup spinach (fresh or frozen)
- 1 bay leaf (crumbled)
- 1 cup coconut milk
- 4 cups vegetable stock
- Salt and pepper to taste
- Herbs for garnish (optional)
- 1/2 cup coconut oil

Directions:

1. In a pressure pot on "sauté" mode, sauté onions and garlic until onions are browned. Once cooked, add the cauliflower and bay leaf and cook for about 5 minutes, stirring occasionally.
2. Add the spinach and continue cooking and stirring for 5 minutes.

3. Pour in the vegetable stock and set the timer for 10 minutes on high pressure to let the mix come to a boil; then allow quick pressure release and add the coconut milk.
4. Season with garnishes of choice as well as salt and pepper. Turn off the pot and mix the soup until it becomes thick and creamy with a hand blender.

Nutrition:

Calories: 114

Total fat: 9g

Saturated fat: 5g

Sodium: 128mg

Carbs: 19g

Fiber: 8g

Protein: 6g

41. Veggie Soup (Pressure- Pot)

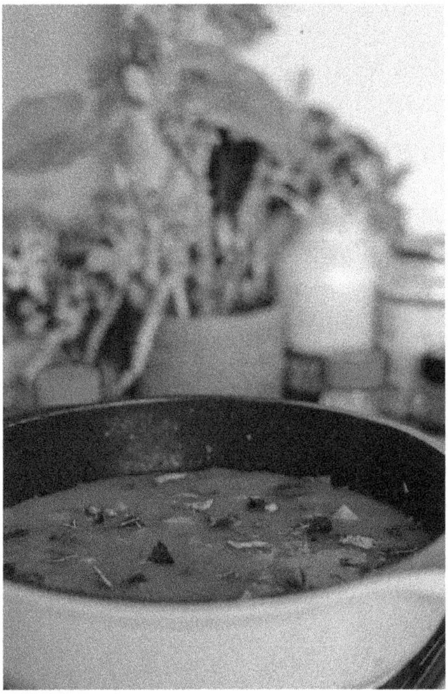

Preparation time: 5 minutes

Cooking time: 10 minutes

Servings: 4

Ingredients:

- 2 tbsp. olive oil

- 1 onion (medium, chopped)
- 3 tbsp. parsley (fresh, minced)
- 1 clove of garlic (minced)
- 3 (14.5 oz.) cans vegetable broth
- 4 cups tomatoes (chopped)
- 1 cup celery (chopped)
- 1 cup carrots (sliced)
- 1 zucchini (halved and sliced)
- 2 tsp. basil (dried, crushed)
- 1/2 tsp. salt
- 1/2 tsp. Italian seasoning
- 1 tsp. red pepper flakes (crushed)
- 5 cups kale leaves (chopped)

Directions:

1. Heat pot on "sauté" mode until it says "hot"; then adds the oil.
2. Attach the onion, and cook until it is tender. Add the parsley and garlic, stirring constantly for 30 seconds; then add the vegetable broth.
3. Stir in the celery, tomato, zucchini, carrots, Italian seasoning, and red pepper to the pot and turn off the heat. Close the lid.
4. Turn the steam option to "sealing," selecting high pressure for 6 minutes. When done, turn the cooker off again, choosing the quick pressure release option; then select "sauté."
5. Add kale, stirring for 3 minutes or so until the soup comes to a boil. Turn the cooker off and serve.

Nutrition:

Calories: 134

Total fat: 9g

Saturated fat: 5g

Sodium: 138mg

Carbs: 26g

Fiber: 8g

Protein: 6g

14 Days Meal Plan For Pegan Diet

Day s	Breakfast	Lunch	Dinner	Dessert
1	BREAKFA ST PALEO MUFFINS	TANGY BROCCOLI SALAD	SWEET POTATO BISQUE	TART APPLE GRANITA
2	PALEO BANANA PANCAKE S	SUMMER ROLLS WITH PEANUT SAUCE	CHICKPEA MEDLEY	LEMON-LIME SHERBET
3	PLANTAI N PANCAKE S	CHEESY WHITE BEAN CAULIFLO WER SOUP	PASTA WITH LEMON AND ARTICHO KES	PAVLOVA WITH PEACHES
4	SWEET POTATO WAFFLES	SPLIT PEA SOUP	ROASTED PINE NUT ORZO	TROPICAL VANILLA SNOW CONE
5	ORANGE AND DATES GRANOL A	QUINOA & CHICKPEA TABBOULE H	BANANA AND ALMOND BUTTER OATS	PEANUT BUTTER, NUT, AND FRUIT COOKIES

6	BREAKFA ST BURRITO	CAULIFLO WER CAESAR SALAD WITH CHICKPEA CROUTONS	RED TOFU CURRY	CHOCOLATE COVERED DATES
7	SPINACH FRITTATA	VEGETABLE ROSE POTATO	SPICY TOMATO-LENTIL STEW	HOT CHOCOLATE
8	SQUASH BLOSSO M FRITTATA	RICE ARUGULA SALAD	MIXED-BEAN CHILI	VANILLA CUPCAKES
9	BREAKFA ST BURGER	TOMATO SALAD	BUTTERN UT SQUASH SOUP	STUFFED DRIED FIGS
10	GREEN BREAKFA ST SMOOTH IE	KALE APPLE ROASTED ROOT VEGETABLE SALAD	SPLIT-PEA SOUP	FETA CHEESECAKE
11	WARM MAPLE AND	RICE ARUGULA SALAD	TOMATO BISQUE	PEAR CROUSTADE

	CINNAMON QUINOA	WITH SESAME GARLIC DRESSING		
12	BLUEBERRY AND CHIA SMOOTHIE	ROASTED LEMON ASPARAGUS WATERCRESS SALAD	CHEESY POTATO-BROCCOLI SOUP	MELOMAKARONA
13	APPLE AND CINNAMON OATMEAL	PUMPKIN AND BRUSSELS SPROUTS MIX	VEGETABLE STEW	LOUKOUMADES (FRIED HONEY BALLS)
14	SPICED ORANGE BREAKFAST COUSCOUS	ALMOND AND TOMATO SALAD	FRIJOLES DE LA OLLA	CRÈME CARAMEL

CPSIA information can be obtained
at www.ICGtesting.com
Printed in the USA
BVHW091036260421
605864BV00003B/411

9 781802 234244